Daily Pregnancy Journey

Due Date

MEDICAL PROFESSIONALS

Obstetrician Gynecologist

Address

Office Number

Doula / Midwife

Address

Office Number

IMPORTANT NUMBERS

Name   Number

DATE _____ / _____ / _____

BREAKFAST

_____
_____
_____
_____

LUNCH

_____
_____
_____
_____

DINNER

_____
_____
_____
_____

SNACKS

_____
_____
_____

H20 INTAKE
8 OZ GLASS

TO DO:
☐ _____
☐ _____
☐ _____

☐ _____
☐ _____
☐ _____
☐ _____
☐ _____

WEIGHT:

PRENATAL VITAMIN ☐

PRENATAL DR. APT:

CRAVINGS

EXERCISE

HOW AM I FEELING?

HRS OF SLEEP / TIME OF DAY

NOTES:

DATE ___ / ___ / ___

BREAKFAST

_____
_____
_____
_____

LUNCH

_____
_____
_____
_____

DINNER

_____
_____
_____
_____

SNACKS

_____
_____

H20 INTAKE
8 OZ GLASS
▽ ▽ ▽ ▽ ▽ ▽ ▽ ▽ ▽ ▽ ▽ ▽

TO DO:
☐ _____
☐ _____
☐ _____

☐ _____
☐ _____
☐ _____
☐ _____
☐ _____

WEIGHT: _____

PRENATAL VITAMIN ☐

PRENATAL DR. APT:

CRAVINGS

EXERCISE

HOW AM I FEELING?

HRS OF SLEEP / TIME OF DAY

NOTES:

DATE _____ / _____ / _____

BREAKFAST

_____
_____
_____
_____
_____

LUNCH

_____
_____
_____
_____
_____

DINNER

_____
_____
_____
_____

SNACKS

_____
_____

H20 INTAKE
8 OZ GLASS

TO DO:
☐ _____   ☐ _____
☐ _____   ☐ _____
☐ _____   ☐ _____
☐ _____   ☐ _____
                    ☐ _____

WEIGHT: _____

PRENATAL VITAMIN ☐

PRENATAL DR. APT: _____

CRAVINGS

EXERCISE

Hi

HOW AM I FEELING?

HRS OF SLEEP / TIME OF DAY

NOTES:

DATE _____ / _____ / _____

BREAKFAST

_____
_____
_____
_____
_____

LUNCH

_____
_____
_____
_____

DINNER

_____
_____
_____
_____

SNACKS

_____
_____

H20 INTAKE
8 OZ GLASS

TO DO:
☐ _____
☐ _____
☐ _____

☐ _____
☐ _____
☐ _____
☐ _____
☐ _____

WEIGHT:

PRENATAL VITAMIN ☐

PRENATAL DR. APT:

CRAVINGS

EXERCISE

HOW AM I FEELING?

HRS OF SLEEP / TIME OF DAY

NOTES:

DATE _____ / _____ / _____

BREAKFAST

_____

_____

_____

_____

_____

_____

LUNCH

_____

_____

_____

_____

_____

DINNER

_____

_____

_____

_____

_____

SNACKS

_____

_____

_____

H20 INTAKE
8 OZ GLASS ∇ ∇ ∇ ∇ ∇ ∇ ∇ ∇ ∇ ∇ ∇ ∇

TO DO:

☐ _____

☐ _____

☐ _____

☐ _____

☐ _____

☐ _____

☐ _____

☐ _____

WEIGHT:

PRENATAL VITAMIN ☐

PRENATAL DR. APT:

CRAVINGS

EXERCISE

HOW AM I FEELING?

HRS OF SLEEP / TIME OF DAY

NOTES:

DATE _____ / _____ / _____

BREAKFAST

_____
_____
_____
_____

LUNCH

_____
_____
_____
_____

DINNER

_____
_____
_____
_____

SNACKS

_____
_____

H20 INTAKE
8 OZ GLASS ▽ ▽ ▽ ▽ ▽ ▽ ▽ ▽ ▽ ▽ ▽ ▽

TO DO:

☐ _____
☐ _____
☐ _____

☐ _____
☐ _____
☐ _____
☐ _____
☐ _____

WEIGHT:

PRENATAL VITAMIN ☐

PRENATAL DR. APT:

CRAVINGS

EXERCISE

HOW AM I FEELING?

HRS OF SLEEP / TIME OF DAY

NOTES:

DATE _____ / _____ / _____

BREAKFAST

_____
_____
_____
_____
_____

LUNCH

_____
_____
_____
_____
_____

DINNER

_____
_____
_____
_____
_____

SNACKS

_____
_____

H20 INTAKE
8 OZ GLASS

TO DO:

☐ _____   ☐ _____
☐ _____   ☐ _____
☐ _____   ☐ _____
☐ _____   ☐ _____
                  ☐ _____

WEIGHT:

PRENATAL VITAMIN ☐

PRENATAL DR. APT:

CRAVINGS

EXERCISE

HOW AM I FEELING?

HRS OF SLEEP / TIME OF DAY

NOTES:

DATE _____ / _____ / _____

BREAKFAST

_____
_____
_____
_____

LUNCH

_____
_____
_____
_____

DINNER

_____
_____
_____
_____

SNACKS

_____
_____

H20 INTAKE
8 OZ GLASS

TO DO:

☐ _____   ☐ _____
☐ _____   ☐ _____
☐ _____   ☐ _____
                   ☐ _____
                   ☐ _____

WEIGHT:

PRENATAL VITAMIN ☐

PRENATAL DR. APT:

CRAVINGS

EXERCISE

HOW AM I FEELING?

HRS OF SLEEP / TIME OF DAY

NOTES:

DATE _____ / _____ / _____

BREAKFAST

LUNCH

DINNER

SNACKS

H20 INTAKE
8 OZ GLASS

TO DO:

- [ ] _____
- [ ] _____
- [ ] _____

- [ ] _____
- [ ] _____
- [ ] _____
- [ ] _____
- [ ] _____

WEIGHT:

PRENATAL VITAMIN [ ]

PRENATAL DR. APT:

CRAVINGS

EXERCISE

HOW AM I FEELING?

HRS OF SLEEP / TIME OF DAY

NOTES:

DATE _____ / _____ / _____

BREAKFAST

LUNCH

DINNER

SNACKS

H20 INTAKE
8 OZ GLASS

TO DO:

☐ _____
☐ _____
☐ _____

☐ _____
☐ _____
☐ _____
☐ _____
☐ _____

WEIGHT:

PRENATAL VITAMIN ☐

PRENATAL DR. APT:

CRAVINGS

EXERCISE

HOW AM I FEELING?

HRS OF SLEEP / TIME OF DAY

NOTES:

DATE _____ / _____ / _____

BREAKFAST

_____
_____
_____
_____
_____

LUNCH

_____
_____
_____
_____

DINNER

_____
_____
_____
_____

SNACKS

_____
_____

H20 INTAKE
8 OZ GLASS

TO DO:

☐ _____
☐ _____
☐ _____

☐ _____
☐ _____
☐ _____
☐ _____
☐ _____

WEIGHT:

PRENATAL VITAMIN ☐

PRENATAL DR. APT:

CRAVINGS

_____

_____

_____

EXERCISE

_____

_____

_____

HOW AM I FEELING?

_____

_____

_____

HRS OF SLEEP / TIME OF DAY

_____

_____

NOTES:

_____

_____

_____

_____

DATE _____ / _____ / _____

BREAKFAST

_____
_____
_____
_____

LUNCH

_____
_____
_____
_____

DINNER

_____
_____
_____
_____

SNACKS

_____
_____

**H20 INTAKE
8 OZ GLASS** ⊔ ⊔ ⊔ ⊔ ⊔ ⊔ ⊔ ⊔ ⊔ ⊔ ⊔ ⊔

TO DO:

☐ _____   ☐ _____
☐ _____   ☐ _____
☐ _____   ☐ _____
                  ☐ _____
                  ☐ _____

WEIGHT:

PRENATAL VITAMIN ☐

PRENATAL DR. APT:

CRAVINGS

EXERCISE

HOW AM I FEELING?

HRS OF SLEEP / TIME OF DAY

NOTES:

DATE _____ / _____ / _____

BREAKFAST

LUNCH

DINNER

SNACKS

H20 INTAKE
8 OZ GLASS

TO DO:

☐ _____
☐ _____
☐ _____

☐ _____
☐ _____
☐ _____
☐ _____
☐ _____

WEIGHT:

PRENATAL VITAMIN ☐

PRENATAL DR. APT:

CRAVINGS

EXERCISE

HOW AM I FEELING?

HRS OF SLEEP / TIME OF DAY

NOTES:

DATE _____ / _____ / _____

BREAKFAST

_____

_____

_____

_____

LUNCH

_____

_____

_____

_____

DINNER

_____

_____

_____

_____

SNACKS

_____

_____

_____

H20 INTAKE
8 OZ GLASS ▽ ▽ ▽ ▽ ▽ ▽ ▽ ▽ ▽ ▽ ▽ ▽

TO DO:
☐ _____   ☐ _____
☐ _____   ☐ _____
☐ _____   ☐ _____
☐ _____   ☐ _____
                        ☐ _____

WEIGHT:

PRENATAL VITAMIN ☐

PRENATAL DR. APT:

CRAVINGS

EXERCISE

HOW AM I FEELING?

HRS OF SLEEP / TIME OF DAY

NOTES:

DATE _____ / _____ / _____

BREAKFAST

_____
_____
_____
_____

LUNCH

_____
_____
_____

DINNER

_____
_____
_____
_____

SNACKS

_____
_____

H20 INTAKE
8 OZ GLASS

TO DO:

☐ _____   ☐ _____
☐ _____   ☐ _____
☐ _____   ☐ _____
                 ☐ _____
                 ☐ _____

WEIGHT:

PRENATAL VITAMIN ☐

PRENATAL DR. APT:

CRAVINGS

EXERCISE

HOW AM I FEELING?

HRS OF SLEEP / TIME OF DAY

NOTES:

BREAKFAST

_____
_____
_____
_____

LUNCH

_____
_____
_____

DINNER

_____
_____
_____
_____

SNACKS

_____
_____

H20 INTAKE
8 OZ GLASS

TO DO:
- [ ] _____
- [ ] _____
- [ ] _____

- [ ] _____
- [ ] _____
- [ ] _____
- [ ] _____
- [ ] _____

WEIGHT:

PRENATAL VITAMIN ☐

PRENATAL DR. APT:

CRAVINGS

EXERCISE

HOW AM I FEELING?

HRS OF SLEEP / TIME OF DAY

NOTES:

DATE _____ / _____ / _____

BREAKFAST

_____

_____

_____

_____

_____

LUNCH

_____

_____

_____

_____

_____

DINNER

_____

_____

_____

_____

SNACKS

_____

_____

H20 INTAKE
8 OZ GLASS

TO DO:

☐ _____
☐ _____
☐ _____

☐ _____
☐ _____
☐ _____
☐ _____
☐ _____

WEIGHT:

PRENATAL VITAMIN ☐

PRENATAL DR. APT:

CRAVINGS

EXERCISE

HOW AM I FEELING?

HRS OF SLEEP / TIME OF DAY

NOTES:

DATE _____ / _____ / _____

BREAKFAST

LUNCH

DINNER

SNACKS

H20 INTAKE
8 OZ GLASS

TO DO:
☐ _____
☐ _____
☐ _____

☐ _____
☐ _____
☐ _____
☐ _____
☐ _____

WEIGHT:

PRENATAL VITAMIN ☐
PRENATAL DR. APT:

CRAVINGS

EXERCISE

HOW AM I FEELING?

HRS OF SLEEP / TIME OF DAY

NOTES:

BREAKFAST

LUNCH

DINNER

SNACKS

H20 INTAKE
8 OZ GLASS

TO DO:

☐ _____
☐ _____
☐ _____

☐ _____
☐ _____
☐ _____
☐ _____
☐ _____

WEIGHT:

PRENATAL VITAMIN ☐

PRENATAL DR. APT:

CRAVINGS

EXERCISE

HOW AM I FEELING?

HRS OF SLEEP / TIME OF DAY

NOTES:

DATE _____ / _____ / _____

BREAKFAST

LUNCH

DINNER

SNACKS

H20 INTAKE
8 OZ GLASS

TO DO:

☐ _____
☐ _____
☐ _____

☐ _____
☐ _____
☐ _____
☐ _____
☐ _____

WEIGHT:

PRENATAL VITAMIN ☐

PRENATAL DR. APT:

CRAVINGS

EXERCISE

HOW AM I FEELING?

HRS OF SLEEP / TIME OF DAY

NOTES:

BREAKFAST

LUNCH

DINNER

SNACKS

H20 INTAKE
8 OZ GLASS

TO DO:

- [ ]
- [ ]
- [ ]

- [ ]
- [ ]
- [ ]
- [ ]
- [ ]

WEIGHT:

PRENATAL VITAMIN [ ]

PRENATAL DR. APT:

CRAVINGS

EXERCISE

HOW AM I FEELING?

HRS OF SLEEP / TIME OF DAY

NOTES:

DATE _____ / _____ / _____

BREAKFAST

_____

_____

_____

_____

_____

LUNCH

_____

_____

_____

_____

DINNER

_____

_____

_____

_____

SNACKS

_____

_____

_____

H20 INTAKE
8 OZ GLASS

TO DO:

☐ _____   ☐ _____

☐ _____   ☐ _____

☐ _____   ☐ _____

☐ _____   ☐ _____

☐ _____

WEIGHT:

PRENATAL VITAMIN ☐

PRENATAL DR. APT:

CRAVINGS

EXERCISE

HOW AM I FEELING?

HRS OF SLEEP / TIME OF DAY

NOTES:

DATE _____ / _____ / _____

BREAKFAST

_____
_____
_____
_____
_____

LUNCH

_____
_____
_____
_____

DINNER

_____
_____
_____
_____

SNACKS

_____
_____

H20 INTAKE
8 OZ GLASS

TO DO:

☐ _____   ☐ _____
☐ _____   ☐ _____
☐ _____   ☐ _____
☐ _____   ☐ _____
                   ☐ _____

WEIGHT:

PRENATAL VITAMIN ☐

PRENATAL DR. APT:

CRAVINGS

EXERCISE

HOW AM I FEELING?

HRS OF SLEEP / TIME OF DAY

NOTES:

DATE _____ / _____ / _____

BREAKFAST
_____
_____
_____
_____
_____

LUNCH
_____
_____
_____
_____

DINNER
_____
_____
_____
_____

SNACKS
_____
_____
_____

H20 INTAKE
8 OZ GLASS

TO DO:
☐ _____
☐ _____
☐ _____

☐ _____
☐ _____
☐ _____
☐ _____
☐ _____

WEIGHT:

PRENATAL VITAMIN ☐

PRENATAL DR. APT:

CRAVINGS

EXERCISE

HOW AM I FEELING?

HRS OF SLEEP / TIME OF DAY

NOTES:

DATE _____ / _____ / _____

BREAKFAST

_____
_____
_____
_____

LUNCH

_____
_____
_____

DINNER

_____
_____
_____

SNACKS

_____
_____

H20 INTAKE
8 OZ GLASS

TO DO:

☐ _____
☐ _____
☐ _____

☐ _____
☐ _____
☐ _____
☐ _____
☐ _____

WEIGHT:

PRENATAL VITAMIN ☐

PRENATAL DR. APT:

CRAVINGS

EXERCISE

HOW AM I FEELING?

HRS OF SLEEP / TIME OF DAY

NOTES:

DATE _____ / _____ / _____

BREAKFAST

_____

_____

_____

_____

LUNCH

_____

_____

_____

_____

DINNER

_____

_____

_____

_____

SNACKS

_____

_____

_____

H20 INTAKE
8 OZ GLASS

TO DO:

☐ _____   ☐ _____
☐ _____   ☐ _____
☐ _____   ☐ _____
                    ☐ _____

WEIGHT:

PRENATAL VITAMIN ☐

PRENATAL DR. APT:

CRAVINGS

EXERCISE

HOW AM I FEELING?

HRS OF SLEEP / TIME OF DAY

NOTES:

DATE _____ / _____ / _____

BREAKFAST

_____
_____
_____
_____

LUNCH

_____
_____
_____
_____

DINNER

_____
_____
_____
_____

SNACKS

_____
_____

H20 INTAKE
8 OZ GLASS

TO DO:

☐ _____
☐ _____
☐ _____

☐ _____
☐ _____
☐ _____
☐ _____
☐ _____

WEIGHT:

PRENATAL VITAMIN ☐

PRENATAL DR. APT:

CRAVINGS

EXERCISE

HOW AM I FEELING?

HRS OF SLEEP / TIME OF DAY

NOTES:

DATE _____ / _____ / _____

BREAKFAST

_____
_____
_____
_____

LUNCH

_____
_____
_____
_____

DINNER

_____
_____
_____
_____

SNACKS

_____
_____

H20 INTAKE
8 OZ GLASS

TO DO:
☐ _____   ☐ _____
☐ _____   ☐ _____
☐ _____   ☐ _____
☐ _____   ☐ _____
                       ☐ _____

WEIGHT:

PRENATAL VITAMIN ☐

PRENATAL DR. APT:

CRAVINGS

EXERCISE

HOW AM I FEELING?

HRS OF SLEEP / TIME OF DAY

NOTES:

DATE _____ / _____ / _____

BREAKFAST

_____
_____
_____
_____
_____

LUNCH

_____
_____
_____
_____
_____

DINNER

_____
_____
_____
_____
_____

SNACKS

_____
_____

H20 INTAKE
8 OZ GLASS

TO DO:

- ☐ _____
- ☐ _____
- ☐ _____

☐ _____
☐ _____
☐ _____
☐ _____

WEIGHT:

PRENATAL VITAMIN ☐

PRENATAL DR. APT:

CRAVINGS

EXERCISE

HOW AM I FEELING?

HRS OF SLEEP / TIME OF DAY

NOTES:

DATE _____ / _____ / _____

BREAKFAST

_____
_____
_____
_____
_____

LUNCH

_____
_____
_____
_____

DINNER

_____
_____
_____
_____

SNACKS

_____
_____

H20 INTAKE
8 OZ GLASS

TO DO:

☐ _____
☐ _____
☐ _____

☐ _____
☐ _____
☐ _____
☐ _____
☐ _____

WEIGHT:

PRENATAL VITAMIN ☐

PRENATAL DR. APT:

CRAVINGS

EXERCISE

HOW AM I FEELING?

HRS OF SLEEP / TIME OF DAY

NOTES:

DATE _____ / _____ / _____

BREAKFAST

_____

_____

_____

_____

LUNCH

_____

_____

_____

_____

DINNER

_____

_____

_____

_____

SNACKS

_____

_____

H20 INTAKE
8 OZ GLASS

TO DO:

☐ _____   ☐ _____
☐ _____   ☐ _____
☐ _____   ☐ _____
                  ☐ _____
                  ☐ _____

WEIGHT:

PRENATAL VITAMIN ☐

PRENATAL DR. APT:

CRAVINGS

EXERCISE

HOW AM I FEELING?

HRS OF SLEEP / TIME OF DAY

NOTES:

DATE _____ / _____ / _____

BREAKFAST

LUNCH

DINNER

SNACKS

H20 INTAKE
8 OZ GLASS

TO DO:

☐ _____

☐ _____

☐ _____

☐ _____

☐ _____

☐ _____

☐ _____

☐ _____

WEIGHT:

PRENATAL VITAMIN ☐

PRENATAL DR. APT:

CRAVINGS

EXERCISE

HOW AM I FEELING?

HRS OF SLEEP / TIME OF DAY

NOTES:

DATE _____ / _____ / _____

BREAKFAST

_____
_____
_____
_____
_____

LUNCH

_____
_____
_____
_____

DINNER

_____
_____
_____
_____

SNACKS

_____
_____

H20 INTAKE
8 OZ GLASS

TO DO:

- ☐ _____
- ☐ _____
- ☐ _____

- ☐ _____
- ☐ _____
- ☐ _____
- ☐ _____
- ☐ _____

WEIGHT:

PRENATAL VITAMIN ☐

PRENATAL DR. APT:

CRAVINGS

EXERCISE

HOW AM I FEELING?

HRS OF SLEEP / TIME OF DAY

NOTES:

DATE _____ / _____ / _____

BREAKFAST

_____
_____
_____
_____
_____

LUNCH

_____
_____
_____
_____

DINNER

_____
_____
_____
_____

SNACKS

_____
_____

H20 INTAKE
8 OZ GLASS

TO DO:

☐ _____   ☐ _____
☐ _____   ☐ _____
☐ _____   ☐ _____
                     ☐ _____
                     ☐ _____

WEIGHT:

PRENATAL VITAMIN ☐

PRENATAL DR. APT:

CRAVINGS

EXERCISE

HOW AM I FEELING?

HRS OF SLEEP / TIME OF DAY

NOTES:

DATE _____ / _____ / _____

BREAKFAST

LUNCH

DINNER

SNACKS

H20 INTAKE
8 OZ GLASS

TO DO:

WEIGHT:

PRENATAL VITAMIN ☐

PRENATAL DR. APT:

CRAVINGS

EXERCISE

HOW AM I FEELING?

HRS OF SLEEP / TIME OF DAY

NOTES:

DATE _____ / _____ / _____

BREAKFAST

_____
_____
_____
_____

LUNCH

_____
_____
_____
_____

DINNER

_____
_____
_____
_____

SNACKS

_____
_____

H20 INTAKE
8 OZ GLASS

TO DO:

☐ _____
☐ _____
☐ _____

☐ _____
☐ _____
☐ _____
☐ _____
☐ _____

WEIGHT:

PRENATAL VITAMIN ☐

PRENATAL DR. APT:

CRAVINGS

EXERCISE

HOW AM I FEELING?

HRS OF SLEEP / TIME OF DAY

NOTES:

BREAKFAST

LUNCH

DINNER

SNACKS

H20 INTAKE
8 OZ GLASS

TO DO:

☐ _____
☐ _____
☐ _____

☐ _____
☐ _____
☐ _____
☐ _____
☐ _____

WEIGHT:

PRENATAL VITAMIN ☐

PRENATAL DR. APT:

CRAVINGS

EXERCISE

HOW AM I FEELING?

HRS OF SLEEP / TIME OF DAY

NOTES:

DATE _____ / _____ / _____

BREAKFAST

_____
_____
_____
_____
_____

LUNCH

_____
_____
_____
_____

DINNER

_____
_____
_____
_____

SNACKS

_____
_____

H20 INTAKE
8 OZ GLASS

TO DO:
☐ _____
☐ _____
☐ _____
☐ _____
☐ _____
☐ _____
☐ _____

WEIGHT:

PRENATAL VITAMIN ☐

PRENATAL DR. APT:

CRAVINGS

EXERCISE

HOW AM I FEELING?

HRS OF SLEEP / TIME OF DAY

NOTES:

DATE _____ / _____ / _____

BREAKFAST

LUNCH

DINNER

SNACKS

H20 INTAKE
8 OZ GLASS

TO DO:
- ☐ _____
- ☐ _____
- ☐ _____

- ☐ _____
- ☐ _____
- ☐ _____
- ☐ _____
- ☐ _____

WEIGHT:

PRENATAL VITAMIN ☐

PRENATAL DR. APT:

CRAVINGS

EXERCISE

HOW AM I FEELING?

HRS OF SLEEP / TIME OF DAY

NOTES:

DATE _____ / _____ / _____

BREAKFAST

_____
_____
_____
_____

LUNCH

_____
_____
_____
_____

DINNER

_____
_____
_____
_____

SNACKS

_____
_____

H20 INTAKE
8 OZ GLASS

TO DO:
- [ ] _____
- [ ] _____
- [ ] _____

- [ ] _____
- [ ] _____
- [ ] _____
- [ ] _____
- [ ] _____

WEIGHT:

PRENATAL VITAMIN ☐

PRENATAL DR. APT:

CRAVINGS

EXERCISE

HOW AM I FEELING?

HRS OF SLEEP / TIME OF DAY

NOTES:

DATE _____ / _____ / _____

BREAKFAST

_____
_____
_____
_____

LUNCH

_____
_____
_____
_____

DINNER

_____
_____
_____
_____

SNACKS

_____
_____

H20 INTAKE
8 OZ GLASS

TO DO:

☐ _____
☐ _____
☐ _____

☐ _____
☐ _____
☐ _____
☐ _____
☐ _____

WEIGHT:

PRENATAL VITAMIN ☐

PRENATAL DR. APT:

CRAVINGS

EXERCISE

HOW AM I FEELING?

HRS OF SLEEP / TIME OF DAY

NOTES:

DATE _____ / _____ / _____

BREAKFAST

_____
_____
_____
_____

LUNCH

_____
_____
_____
_____

DINNER

_____
_____
_____
_____

SNACKS

_____
_____

H20 INTAKE
8 OZ GLASS

TO DO:

☐ _____
☐ _____
☐ _____

☐ _____
☐ _____
☐ _____
☐ _____

WEIGHT:

PRENATAL VITAMIN ☐

PRENATAL DR. APT:

CRAVINGS

EXERCISE

HOW AM I FEELING?

HRS OF SLEEP / TIME OF DAY

NOTES:

DATE _____ / _____ / _____

BREAKFAST

LUNCH

DINNER

SNACKS

H20 INTAKE
8 OZ GLASS

TO DO:
- [ ] _____
- [ ] _____
- [ ] _____

- [ ] _____
- [ ] _____
- [ ] _____
- [ ] _____

WEIGHT:

PRENATAL VITAMIN [ ]

PRENATAL DR. APT:

CRAVINGS

EXERCISE

HOW AM I FEELING?

HRS OF SLEEP / TIME OF DAY

NOTES:

DATE _____ / _____ / _____

BREAKFAST

_____

_____

_____

_____

LUNCH

_____

_____

_____

_____

DINNER

_____

_____

_____

_____

SNACKS

_____

_____

H20 INTAKE
8 OZ GLASS ▽ ▽ ▽ ▽ ▽ ▽ ▽ ▽ ▽ ▽ ▽ ▽

TO DO:

☐ _____   ☐ _____
☐ _____   ☐ _____
☐ _____   ☐ _____
                   ☐ _____
                   ☐ _____

WEIGHT:

PRENATAL VITAMIN ☐

PRENATAL DR. APT:

CRAVINGS

EXERCISE

HOW AM I FEELING?

HRS OF SLEEP / TIME OF DAY

NOTES:

DATE _____ / _____ / _____

BREAKFAST

_____
_____
_____
_____

LUNCH

_____
_____
_____
_____

DINNER

_____
_____
_____
_____

SNACKS

_____
_____

H20 INTAKE
8 OZ GLASS

TO DO:

☐ _____   ☐ _____
☐ _____   ☐ _____
☐ _____   ☐ _____
                 ☐ _____
                 ☐ _____

WEIGHT:

PRENATAL VITAMIN ☐

PRENATAL DR. APT:

CRAVINGS

EXERCISE

HOW AM I FEELING?

HRS OF SLEEP / TIME OF DAY

NOTES:

DATE _____ / _____ / _____

BREAKFAST

_____
_____
_____
_____

LUNCH

_____
_____
_____
_____

DINNER

_____
_____
_____
_____

SNACKS

_____
_____

H20 INTAKE
8 OZ GLASS

TO DO:

☐ _____   ☐ _____
☐ _____   ☐ _____
☐ _____   ☐ _____
☐ _____   ☐ _____
               ☐ _____

WEIGHT:

PRENATAL VITAMIN ☐

PRENATAL DR. APT:

CRAVINGS

EXERCISE

HOW AM I FEELING?

HRS OF SLEEP / TIME OF DAY

NOTES:

DATE _____ / _____ / _____

BREAKFAST

_____
_____
_____
_____

LUNCH

_____
_____
_____
_____

DINNER

_____
_____
_____
_____

SNACKS

_____
_____
_____

H20 INTAKE
8 OZ GLASS

TO DO:

☐ _____ ☐ _____
☐ _____ ☐ _____
☐ _____ ☐ _____
☐ _____ ☐ _____
             ☐ _____

WEIGHT:

PRENATAL VITAMIN ☐

PRENATAL DR. APT:

CRAVINGS

EXERCISE

HOW AM I FEELING?

HRS OF SLEEP / TIME OF DAY

NOTES:

DATE _____ / _____ / _____

BREAKFAST

_____
_____
_____
_____
_____

LUNCH

_____
_____
_____
_____

DINNER

_____
_____
_____
_____

SNACKS

_____
_____

H20 INTAKE
8 OZ GLASS

TO DO:
☐ _____
☐ _____
☐ _____

☐ _____
☐ _____
☐ _____
☐ _____
☐ _____

WEIGHT:

PRENATAL VITAMIN ☐

PRENATAL DR. APT:

CRAVINGS

EXERCISE

HOW AM I FEELING?

HRS OF SLEEP / TIME OF DAY

NOTES:

DATE _____ / _____ / _____

BREAKFAST

LUNCH

DINNER

SNACKS

H20 INTAKE
8 OZ GLASS

TO DO:

☐ _____
☐ _____
☐ _____

☐ _____
☐ _____
☐ _____
☐ _____
☐ _____

WEIGHT:

PRENATAL VITAMIN ☐

PRENATAL DR. APT:

CRAVINGS

EXERCISE

HOW AM I FEELING?

HRS OF SLEEP / TIME OF DAY

NOTES:

DATE _____ / _____ / _____

BREAKFAST

_____
_____
_____
_____

LUNCH

_____
_____
_____
_____

DINNER

_____
_____
_____
_____

SNACKS

_____
_____

H20 INTAKE
8 OZ GLASS

TO DO:

☐ _____
☐ _____
☐ _____

☐ _____
☐ _____
☐ _____
☐ _____
☐ _____

WEIGHT:

PRENATAL VITAMIN ☐

PRENATAL DR. APT:

CRAVINGS

EXERCISE

HOW AM I FEELING?

HRS OF SLEEP / TIME OF DAY

NOTES:

Made in the USA
Las Vegas, NV
05 December 2021

36146700R00057